Empowered to Birth Naturally:

One Woman's Journey to Homebirth

By Patrice A. London

DISCLAIMER

This book details the author's personal experiences with and opinions about birth. The author is not a healthcare provider.

The author and publisher are providing this book and its contents on an "as is" basis and make no representations or warranties of any kind with respect to this book or its contents. The author and publisher disclaim all such representations and warranties, including for example warranties of merchantability and healthcare for a particular purpose. In addition, the author and publisher do not represent or warrant that the information accessible via this book is accurate, complete or current.

The statements made about products and services have not been evaluated by the U.S. Food and Drug Administration. They are not intended to diagnose, treat, cure, or prevent any condition or disease. Please consult with your own physician or healthcare specialist regarding the suggestions and recommendations made in this book.

Except as specifically stated in this book, neither the author or

Dedication

To my Granddaddy, Reverend Samuel A. Johnson, Sr.: You were much more than just my grandfather. I miss you...

To my children Jaiela, Jenai and Jasmine: You are my greatest and most fulfilling work yet!

Acknowledgements

Thank you Jesus!

To my husband, Jermaine: Thank you for pushing me. You are my everything and more...

To my mother, Teri Brown: Thank you for loving me, respecting me, and being my best friend

To my sister-cousin, Tami Hawkins : Thank you! You add more to my life than you'll ever know.

To my sister-friends Orieyama Linebarger and Tori Ervin, thank you for your continued friendship, support, and honoring me by attending my first homebirth!

Tori you took some amazing pictures!

To my editor, Cindy Fleming-Wood, you are awesome! Thank you so much!

To my uncle, Martin Johnson: I'm so blessed to have you! Thank you for taking up where Granddad left off.

Nikole Jones: Nik the cover is beautiful! Thank you for bringing my vision to life!

Angela at Booklocker.com: You rock lady!

Additionally, I thank Todd at Booklocker, my uncle, Frank Johnson, and all who encouraged me along the way when I was doubtful such a book needed to materialize. You helped make this possible.

Contents

Introduction 1

My First (Hospital) Birth 7

My Second (Birth Center) Birth 15

Miscarriage 23

Home Sweet Homebirth! 25

Interviews of Birth Attendees 39

My Final Thoughts 61

Homebirth Photos 63

About the Author 105

Introduction

In our society, when starting new adventures people tend to pay close attention to detail. When considering buying a house, going to college, getting married, and even buying a television, people conduct extensive research. This same care and attention to detail is all but forgotten when it comes to the life-changing process of giving birth. This area is all too often left to the "experts." This shouldn't be the case. If more people would research the current medical model of care and the midwifery model of care, the results could be revolutionary. More women just might begin to trust that their bodies can, in fact, do what they were created to do — and do it well.

Of course, some don't consider the *how* of giving birth to be important. They just want the end result — a healthy baby. We assume that the medical profession has our best interests at heart when various interventions are doled out "for the benefit of mother and baby." There is no consideration of any long-term effects those interventions may have on mother and baby. It's all just accepted. Then, our society wonders why the cesarean rates are climbing. I believe the *how* of giving birth is of the utmost importance. I believe one can have the end result and a whole lot more. I've experienced firsthand how life-changing the process of birth can be. I've experienced it in a negative and positive light and would like to share those experiences with you.

It is not my intent to imply that homebirth is for everyone. My hope is, however, that every woman will seek to take birth back and make it her own. I would love to see women educated concerning the intricacies of pregnancy and childbirth and, therefore, making informed decisions concerning the way they govern themselves throughout pregnancy — even before pregnancy when possible — and especially in preparation for, and during, childbirth.

All too often, people are very close-minded about what they don't understand or know anything about. Of course, the lack of knowledge doesn't preclude one from making ridiculously callous, crude, and plain ignorant comments. I've heard far too many references to homebirth in particular that are utterly unfounded and just wrong. The fact is, the medical model that so many have bought into is the *newbie*, not homebirth. Ever since the medical model was introduced, the rates of cesareans and many other interventions have increased drastically and steadily. The old adage, "If it ain't broke, don't fix it," certainly applies here. Even with all of the evidence, people remain as ignorant as ever concerning unmedicated birth. What's even more incredulous is that the very people who declare it unsafe or unnecessary have *never* experienced or attended an unmedicated or homebirth.

I must preface the following pages by saying that although it is obvious that I have very strong feelings concerning those I've come in contact with in the medical model of childbirth, I do not undermine the necessity of the profession. Obstetricians and gynecologists are most definitely needed. I am especially grateful when I consider my cousin Tami's experience in giving birth to her first child, Jordynn. Because of the care and expertise the doctor brought at the end of her pregnancy, Tami and Jordynn are alive and thriving today.

The problem arises, however, when that same care one receives out of necessity during an emergency, becomes routine. Normal labor and birth should not be seen as a problem to be fixed or a disease to be cured. The same care Tami received in her urgent situation becomes an intrusive, unnecessary, hindrance and is sometimes even harmful in a normal, low-risk birth. When Tami neared her expected due date with her second daughter, Kennedy, she was denied the right to even try for a vaginal birth simply because she had a cesarean with her first.

All too often it is difficult for a woman wishing to have an unmedicated birth in the hospital to achieve that goal. I would like to see that change. The pregnant women themselves should be educated and ultimately in charge of this process.

One either views birth as a medical event or a natural process. Unfortunately, mainstream thinking leads most to believe it is a medical event. It's no wonder with the images portrayed in the media. Birth is too often seen as an urgent, chaotic, and scary event that only doctors are able to handle. Television shows dramatize it by showing panic-ridden women and their loved ones in utter chaos. A woman is completely fine one moment; then, suddenly her water breaks and she's instantly experiencing the most crippling pain she's ever experienced in her life. Then you later see doctors scrambling into the hospital room screaming, "Push!" We are constantly bombarded with these scenes of tumultuous confusion that all too often end with sudden decisions to perform cesareans. It's no wonder women are fearful and have trouble trusting the process.

Choosing to give birth at home had nothing to do with wanting to be old fashioned. The idea didn't stem from any sort of feminist "I am woman hear me roar" views. I don't like pain any more than the next rationally sane individual. Simply put, I view birth as a natural process that is to be respected, awed, and pretty much left alone. Choosing to give birth at home is more about the fact that I have complete faith in my body and its ability to bring forth my babies. Moreover, I have faith in the God who made my body. I know He has equipped me to be able to give birth and enjoy it. Birth can be a wonderfully empowering experience. I've been blessed to be able to experience birth this way twice. My first birth proved to be a catalyst for more education, better parenting practices, and subsequently, more enjoyable births in the future.

For me, a wonderful birthing experience does not happen in a hospital. It happens in the sanctity of my own home. Because of my second and third birth experiences, I am able to look back at my births with a contented smile and sigh. They were absolutely wonderful!

I am grateful that you have picked up my book. In the following pages, I will share my experiences, good and bad, and how I made the journey from a hospital to a birth center and, finally, a homebirth. It is my hope that something within these pages causes you to think differently concerning birth.

My First (Hospital) Birth

My first birth had a horrible impact on me; so horrible, I vowed that things would be different in subsequent births.

I approached birth believing that my body was made to give birth, so I didn't see a need for medication. I am far more afraid of the medicine routinely given, and possible reactions to them on me and my baby, than of just going through the motions of labor and being done once the baby is born. I was 21 years old and very excited to be able to give birth naturally (with no medication). I had written out my birth plan as I was instructed by my doctor and Lamaze instructor. If I had known better, I would have never experienced a hospital birth at all.

I believe hospitals are for the sick and not the best place for a person with a low-risk pregnancy to give birth. It's all an assembly line/money making situation for them and I'd rather not be a part of that.

Looking back, my birth plan for my first birth was quite simple; I wanted no medication, and I wanted to push in a squatting position so that gravity would help me out. My husband and I have big heads so I figured our children are destined to follow suit — and so far, they haven't disappointed.

The first thing they did when I got to my room in the hospital was attach me to IVs and force me to lie on my back — *the worst position ever for a laboring mom.* You'd think they know this, since it's their profession, but it's not about the mom or the baby; it's about what's best for the hospital staff and their ability to monitor things easily and get you out as quickly as possible. The quicker they can get one out, the quicker they can get another in. I wasn't allowed to even go to the bathroom and, frankly, didn't feel the sensation because they gave me pain medication to make me sleep off and on. Not allowing me to urinate prolonged my labor tremendously. (Another thing one would think they'd be privy to, being that it's their profession.)

Eventually one of the nurses came in and realized I'd not urinated once the entire time. At that point I was catheterized and guess what? I progressed quickly and was soon ready to push – or so I was told. Because of the pain medication I'd been given, I couldn't feel the urge to push.

Suddenly, everyone began screaming at me to push and as I pushed, they'd count. Now, my Lamaze coach always said, "Never push past 10 because the flow of oxygen to the baby will become restricted and they'll have to give you an oxygen mask." So with everyone yelling and prompting me to push, I began to push; someone started counting and, when they got to 10, I stopped. The baby's head, which was crowning went back in. I tried to sit up (remember, my plan was to squat) and I was pushed back down on my back and told to keep pushing until they told me to stop. After a few times of my refusing to go past 10 and the baby's head playing peek-a-boo, I decided to try it their way because this *is* an assembly line situation to them. And, I didn't want them to suddenly declare that my pelvis was too small to give birth vaginally or that the baby was in distress and prepare me for a cesarean. So I pushed on my back way past 10 and what do you know, someone screamed, "The baby needs oxygen!" They whipped out the oxygen mask. I tried again to sit up and was pushed back down and told to push more. After a while the doctor got out a vacuum extractor and "assisted me" by pulling my baby's head out as I pushed. My little cone-head baby girl, Jaiela, was born on Memorial Day (5/25/1998) at 2:24 p.m., weighing in at 6lbs 12oz, but not until after I was ripped because of the force of the vacuum extractor and the impatient doctor who wouldn't let me sit up and allow gravity to help get the baby out.

At this point I was livid but completely vulnerable and at the mercy of the hospital staff. They took Jaiela to the other side of the room to clean and check her. The doctor then told me he had to stitch me up because I was ripped (wonder why?). He gave me a shot down there and immediately began stitching me up. I admit I have a high tolerance for pain but I was so sick of this man by then that I yelled, "I'm feeling this!" After having him poke me all around my vaginal area with that needle over and over to numb me, he began to stitch me up again. My mom and husband looked highly annoyed at the callous way the doctor handled me. It was obvious that I could still feel every bit of the stitching process. I simply resigned, "Forget it!" I've not felt the numbing effects of the needle yet.

What's worse is that when he stitched me up, he did something very wrong. Days after the birth I kept smelling something funky. At first I thought maybe it was a normal part of having a baby but I got a mirror and looked anyway. There was some fleshy pink skin left simply hanging out. I later had to go to my ob/gyn to have it removed with a shot of something that burned it off. Needless to say, it was very weird and painful.

By the time I was able to hold and see Jaiela for the first time, I must say after 33 ½ hours of mostly unproductive, excruciating pain, I was not impressed. I didn't cry tears of joy and feel all lovey-dovey. I was just angry, ridiculously tired, and I thought my baby looked funny.

I was in such a lethargic state after the birth that I embarrassed my poor step-father and uncle. What's funny is I don't remember every detail but when my mom recalled it; I must say I can't deny its occurrence. My step-father and uncle were allowed to come into the room not too long after I'd had the baby. I remember them standing at the foot of my bed smiling and then suddenly leaving not too long after. My mom said that after a while, the iced pad that a nurse put under my bottom must have begun to irritate me because all of a sudden, I took it off and threw the bloody pad — which landed near the feet of my step-father and uncle. Not exactly one of my best, moments I must admit.

Because of the sleeping medication they gave me during labor, Jaiela slept in a weird, drug-like state the entire 3 days that I spent in the hospital. She wouldn't even wake up to eat. The nurses further annoyed me by coming in every 2 hours trying to force Jaiela to breastfeed. A lactation consultant came in once to help us. She came in, and without uttering a single word, snatched my breast and tried to force it into Jaiela's mouth. She was not easily awakened, and because of this, I never learned to nurse properly while in the hospital and had problems in the weeks to come.

Jaiela and I worked it out in the end and went on to continue breastfeeding well past her first birthday.

I hate that her birth was so terrible. As long as I can help it by having a healthy pregnancy, that will never happen again. People often tell me I'm brave when they hear of my birth center and homebirth but I think they're the ones who are brave, entrusting such a personal and powerful experience to strangers who don't always have you or your baby's best interest at heart.

Birth shouldn't be rushed as if going through a drive-thru. What is popular/mainstream is not always best. Most who have gone through labor in a more mainstream way cannot imagine it, but I actually *enjoyed* my second and third births and, God-willing, plan to enjoy a fourth as well...

My Second (Birth Center) Birth

This one was good — well, not completely good. I hated the ride to the birth center. I think it's horrible to have to ride anywhere when you're smack dab in the middle of labor land. The last thing one wants during labor is a bumpy ride in the car.

The entire labor from start to finish wasn't even 3 hours.

Before I became pregnant again I'd done my research. I decided I wanted to have a homebirth for my subsequent births. The problem was, when I did become pregnant again, we were living with my mom and she wasn't at all pleased with the idea.

When I told my mom and husband I wanted them both present when I conducted my interview with a midwife, they freaked. "You want to have a baby where?!" So after a heated discussion with me yelling, "I'm the one who has to give birth to this child! I'm not sick! I'm pregnant and I'm *not* going through another hospital birth!" We compromised on the next best thing, a birth center birth.

The world of midwifery was new and exciting and I was an absolute sponge, soaking up every part of the whole experience. It was nothing like my doctor visits during my previous pregnancy. You know how one typically spends more time in the waiting room than in the actual visit with the doctor? Well, it was the opposite with the four midwives rotating this particular birth center. They were so thorough that I left that experience knowing far more than the average person knows about pregnancy and birth.

I think most of all the difference between my midwives and doctors was the love and respect I felt whenever in their presence. Even now, the difference is amazing. I was a part of the whole process, not merely a patient having things done to me. They never tried to impose anything on me but gave me all the information I needed in order to make more informed choices throughout my pregnancy and during labor. It was mine to do with as I pleased, which was a refreshing contrast to my previous pregnancy and birth.

Being a stay-at-home, homeschooling mom meant that my then 4-year-old was with me during each visit. She was not only welcomed by my midwives, but she was sought after to help with monitoring the baby's heartbeat. She was able to be actively involved every step of the way. It was only natural that she'd be present at the birth and, with the help of my cousin Tami who was also present, cut her sister's umbilical cord once she was born.

My mucous plug came out on July 3rd so I knew that labor would begin soon.

I went into labor at about 2:40 a.m. on July 4th and, as always, my mom was the one who stayed up with me. My mom was there for my last labor and she stayed up with me the whole time. My hubby couldn't handle it and was knocked out until just about time for me to push. So, this time, we decided not to even awaken anyone until it was time to go to the birth center.

I called my midwife to let her know that I thought active labor had begun. I wasn't sure because, unlike my first labor, the pain just wasn't that bad at all. Since then, I've learned that the synthetic version of what a woman's body produces naturally during labor can make labor pains not only stronger, but less effective. I know this to be true because my second and third births weren't nearly as painful as the first.

I was advised to call my midwife back when my contractions were at least 5 minutes apart consecutively for an hour. My mom kept track of the contractions while I moved about, going to the bathroom occasionally, bathing, and just laboring. An hour later, my mom called the midwife to tell her that my contractions were about a minute, or less, apart so she told us to meet her at the birth center in about an hour.

I remember feeling that the time to push was close and without trying to push, could actually feel the baby's head bulging out and going back during contractions. I thought about my wanting to have a homebirth anyway and wasn't at all afraid of the prospect of possibly giving birth at home.

We woke up my husband, daughter Jaiela, and cousin Tami, and prepared to leave for the birth center, totally forgetting the baby's car seat. Thankfully the birth center was only about 7 minutes from the house. Unfortunately we also forgot to bring a camera so we have no pictures of any part of this birth.

On the way, my husband was able to run red lights and, though he liked that part of it, he was deathly afraid because I told him I could feel the head crowning with each contraction. He thought I was going to give birth in the car! I could have slapped him because it seemed as if he ran over every pothole DC had to offer!

We arrived at the birth center at exactly 5 a.m. My midwife and Tami were on either side of me, helping me as I tried to run to the birthing room in between contractions. The contractions were way too strong for me to walk, talk, or do anything but breathe through at that point and, oddly enough, it still wasn't nearly as painful as my first birth. This was the point during my first (hospital) birth where my husband says I begged for an epidural! It never crossed my mind with my second or third births, which is great since they didn't have one available anyway.

As soon as I got to the room, my mom laughed at me because she said I hurriedly snatched off and threw my panties across the room. She said she was sure I had some kind of Velcro panties on. When you are in labor, you are not at all modest. I couldn't have cared less about people seeing me naked.

My midwife asked if she could check my cervix and, as I suspected, I was fully dilated, completely effaced, and ready to push. She didn't scream in my face to get me to push though. No one did. She simply looked at me, smiled, and said, "Whenever, you're ready..."

For the most part, when I'm in pain, I clam up. I can't scream or talk or anything. I am still aware of what's happening around me but have trouble communicating. At some point while pushing I let out what sounded like a primitive, guttural moan. My then 5-year-old climbed onto the bed with me. My mom thought it was too much for her and wanted to take her out of the room, but I got up the strength to speak and told her no. I'd prepared my daughter for it. My mom stayed put and my daughter continued to climb onto the bed and she began rubbing my head. That was a magical moment for me, one that I couldn't have experienced in a hospital. I'm telling you, the moment she touched my head and our eyes met, all the pain that I felt at that moment completely vanished. I couldn't believe it. As long as I focused on her innocent and caring face, I felt nothing but painless contractions that resembled flexing muscles. That was a moment I'll never forget. I planned to maximize on that during my next labor.

Throughout labor, it never occurred to me that my water never broke. When I had Jaiela, the doctors broke my water. With Jenai, everything was left intact. The contrast in care still astonishes me today. Ideas and procedures that are deemed necessary in one setting are completely abandoned in another.

Then, 18 minutes after arriving at the birth center, I gave birth to my second little girl who was immediately laid next to me. She was born in the caul (in the bag, with her bag of waters intact) at 7 lb 6 oz, almost a whole pound larger than my first and I wasn't ripped. I remember seeing what appeared to be a look of recognition on her face when we looked at one another. It was as if she knew who I was. I thought she looked exactly like my recently deceased grandfather. Tami then helped Jaiela cut the umbilical cord. It was wonderful.

All I was required to do before leaving the birth center was to bathe, breastfeed, eat, and urinate and I could go home. So by 9:45 a.m. on July 4th, I was back at home, able to enjoy the holiday with my family and friends who came over. And, best of all, I was able to enjoy the holiday with my new baby.

I remember my midwife looking at me and the baby before we left the birth center. She told me that I'd done very well and said, "Next time, have your baby at home." My plan was to do just that.

Miscarriage

In May of 2006, I discovered I was pregnant again, only to experience heartache after miscarrying the child days after the discovery. Everything happened so fast that, at times, I questioned whether it was all real. During this time, I discovered the lack of support for a woman who experiences this type of loss. A life is lost but there's not much that happens in the way of closure and, frankly, people are all too often insensitive about it. In a sorry attempt to help, they tell a hurting mother that it just wasn't meant to be, the baby is in a better place or, "You're young, you can have more."

I think the worst part of the experience for me was when the whole situation was completely dismissed by one doctor.

When I visited this doctor, the first thing she said was that I had protein in my urine and that's how I got a false positive. She hadn't even checked my urine! When I told her that I had tested positive with a few different tests before going on to have an unusually painful and heavy cycle, she asked pointedly, "Would you really want to know every time your body aborted a fetus?" Stunned, I looked her square in the eyes and replied emphatically, "Yes I would! I would never want to be aloof concerning what goes on with my body!" I left her office and never went back. How many other women has she dismissed that way? How dare she? Some may scoff at the idea of wanting to know but my thinking is that perhaps, if my body did this a number of times, I could assist my doctor in diagnosing and fixing a possible problem in my reproductive system that would otherwise go undetected.

Home Sweet Homebirth!

When I became pregnant again 4 months after miscarrying, I started to bleed a little at about 7 weeks. My midwife, Anne, advised me to go to the emergency room just to make sure everything was fine. While being examined, the doctor asked for my ob/gyn's name. I told him that I was seeing a midwife and gave her name. He then asked where in New Jersey her office was located. When I told him she was in New York, he stopped and asked sarcastically, "So, when you go into labor, you're going to travel all the way to New York?" I replied succinctly, "No, she'll come to me, I'm having a homebirth." He then stated, "You're looking for trouble." He then sent me home with conflicting reports. He said that I could possibly lose the baby but the results of the sonogram showed a normal heart rate and HCG levels in the baby denoting everything in working order. And it was. I am sometimes tempted to send him a card with a picture of my family all huddled around the birthing tub, minutes after the birth, admiring our new baby.

This time around I interviewed and chose a holistic midwife. I enjoyed the holistic side of it all. I learned how to eat better and one thing that stuck with me was the glucose test. Rather than drink that nasty soda type of sugar-laden drink, I was on a restrictive diet for 3 days and on the day of the test, I drank grape juice. That was very interesting. I learned that some glucose tests that come back positive come back that way because the soda drink is filled with sugar. That makes no sense to give such a drink if it can cause false positives!

When planning a homebirth, one has to also plan for possible complications as well. We had directions to the hospital posted on the refrigerator in the event they were needed. My midwife works with a doctor who specializes in high-risk pregnancies. I met with him beforehand so that, in the event that I'd have to be transferred to the hospital with complications, we'd already be acquainted. This doctor was absolutely wonderful. He spoke of his experiences watching his now deceased mother who was a midwife. He, unlike the other doctors I'd dealt with, applauded my decision to give birth at home and was more than happy to be my back-up physician if I needed to be transported to the hospital. It was nice to meet such a doctor. I felt confident, as did he and my midwife, that I'd not have to see him again but if I did, I felt just as confident that I would be in great hands if complications arose.

With all our bases covered, I could go on with the business of growing my baby and enjoying my pregnancy.

When I'd progressed to about 33 weeks or so, I began to shop for my list of items needed for the homebirth. My midwife would come with her bags of course but there were items that I was responsible for supplying as well. I had all kinds of things like gloves, a bowl for the placenta, many receiving blankets, aluminum foil, Chux pads for catching fluids, and a whole lot more. The list was long and a lot of fun to shop for. When most people think of homebirth they picture a chaotic scene with blood and fluids splattered everywhere. It's not like that at all. I'd planned to have a water birth and rented an aquadoula birthing tub. As the time got closer to my expected due date, I lined my bed with several layers. Against my mattress was an inexpensive flannel-back table cloth, followed by a set of old sheets. On top of that was another flannel-back table cloth and another set of old sheets. This was done several times so that if I had soiled my bed at any time, the soiled layer could be easily peeled away to reveal another clean, already made bed.

Because we wanted to be surprised with the sex of the baby this time around, I opted to not get another sonogram. I didn't want to accidentally see or hear anything. However, between 38 and 39 weeks, I'd had a big weight gain and my midwife was concerned. We thought that either the baby was a huge frog baby with legs spread open on both sides of my womb or there were two babies! I went in for a sonogram to be sure and was ready to pass out when the technician said, "8 lb 14 oz." I thought to myself, "I'm going to give birth to a toddler!" I'm 4' 10" and at first I freaked out. Then I remembered a cousin who is small who had a few 8-lb babies and was just fine. I figured if she could handle it, I could too. When I called my midwife to report the size of the baby she gasped, then said that although the sonogram could be off a bit, in order to prevent too much more growth, I was to eliminate sugar from my diet for the remainder of my pregnancy. I was fine with that as I instinctively knew I'd give birth a few days later anyway.

Sure enough, as we drove to a ceremony involving my two older daughters, mild labor pains began. Like my second labor,

I wasn't sure if it was real because even though it was enough for me to take notice, it wasn't really bad. I called my midwife who told me to begin monitoring the contractions and let her know when they were worse.

In addition to my mom who traveled from Washington, DC, I invited two dear friends, Tori and Orieyama, to be a part of the birth. Tori lived about a 20-minute drive away from me; while Orie lived in Maryland and would have about a 3 ½ hour drive to get here. I treasure both ladies and the impact they've had on my life. We went to high school together. And, though there were times — years even — when we weren't in contact, once we'd reconnect, we always picked up right where we left off.

Even after my family moved over 200 miles away, my relationship with Orie continued to grow.

When I first began to feel labor pains on a Wednesday, I called her and she was at my door within hours. Of course my labor didn't progress, so on Friday morning around 4 or 5 a.m., she drove back home, went to work, and drove 3 1/2 hours back to New Jersey after work. She must have been exhausted, not to mention the gas and tolls she paid, but she never complained.

After going through contraction after contraction and not progressing any further, I called my midwife Friday morning and asked if we could induce labor naturally. I was approaching 39 weeks and didn't want to carry the baby too much longer with her being so big and possibly getting bigger. A few hours later I was at her office. Our plan was two-fold: 1) Sweeping the membranes and 2) ingesting a 4-oz solution consisting of 2 oz of vodka and 2 oz of castor oil every hour for up to 3 hours. I went into her office having dilated only 1 cm and left at about – 3 to 4 cm.

Being home and laboring was wonderful. It was nice to be able to move how, when, and where I wanted and not have to leave for an uncomfortable ride in the car. Labor is hard enough work without being confined to any one space and having to travel at the height of it.

Before things got rough, we went to a store and walked around a bit. I was so large, I was often asked about my due date. The associate at the store asked me and when I told her I was in labor at that moment; she smiled, and hurried me out the store!

After returning home, my then 3-year old daughter, Jenai, and I used a sheet and tied it around my neck and under my belly using the rebozo technique. This was to assist the baby with getting in an optimal position for decent into the birth canal. I walked around in my backyard looking at wild mushrooms with Jenai. Then I decided to try "dancing the baby down". That was fun! We turned on some music and partied hard, well as hard as I could anyway. A few hours later, I decided to go on to try the castor oil. Yuck!!! I threw up the castor oil and vodka mixture immediately. I'm not a drinker at all. So, I decided to trade in the vodka for orange juice. Though it was still horrific, I was able to keep it down. A few hours later, my labor began to progress. I was thrilled. I was about to have my first homebirth and meet my new baby!

At this point, I'm not sure if I'd opt to induce again. Part of me can't help but wonder when I would have given birth if I'd waited for things to progress naturally. At the time, I was more afraid of the baby being so big that I could possibly need a cesarean. That was my greatest fear when I heard the baby's size.

Soon after, Orie came back with another friend Dana; my labor began to progress. We all sat around talking. I spoke with my midwife every so often to update her. I used my labor ball to help ease the pain in my back and was just enjoying my company. Eventually, my daughters went to bed. We told them we'd wake them up when it was time for the birth. My contractions quickly got to a point where I couldn't easily talk through them so I called Tori and my midwife and told them to come.

Here's where my awareness of time left. I remember my husband going upstairs with me to help me take a shower. I didn't want to be funky for the birth and thought the water would help ease the contractions. My contractions really began to move along and I was slowly but surely slipping into labor land. This is where you hear what's going on around you, but you're kind of not there. You're somewhere far, far away. While in the shower, I tried to grab something to brace myself through a contraction but there was nothing to grab! I got out and sat on the toilet for a moment and another contraction started. I reached out to grab something again in order to brace myself but again there was nothing to grab! At this moment my husband who was kneeling in front of me kissed me. It was the sweetest and most perfect thing to do at that moment. When we kissed, I felt no pain at all. He was my epidural. I will never forget that moment. At a time when most men would be oblivious as to their place or what to do, he stopped thinking, allowed instinct to take over, and did the perfect thing at the perfect moment, making my first homebirth that much more memorable.

Soon after, I went to my bed and labored there for a while. This was around the time when my midwife, doula, and girlfriend Tori arrived. I don't think I bothered to put on any clothes after leaving the bathroom and remember someone covering me once I got to my bed. I admit, I'm not the most modest person but all modesty was completely tossed aside while I was in labor. It was the farthest thing from my mind. At this point my hormones began to go crazy and I became extremely cold, then extremely hot. Then I gingerly announced to no one in particular that I was going to throw up and my wonderful doula picked up a nearby trash can just in time to catch it.

After a while, I moved downstairs into my living room area and onto a couch where I did the bulk of my laboring. I wanted to be close to the aquadoula tub that was just a few steps from the couch. I continued for a while to go from hot to cold. During one of those moments someone placed a wet rag on my forehead. At the point where I became unbearably hot, I took the towel off my head and threw it almost hitting Orie, while everyone got a good chuckle.

Remembering how moaning helped me at the end of my last labor, I began to moan through my contractions as they got harder and harder. I'm a coloratura soprano which is the highest soprano voice. I probably sounded more like a bass that night with my low, guttural moaning.

In between contractions, I'd somehow sleep. I remember a nurse telling me when I was in the hospital laboring with my firstborn, to try and rest in between contractions. I thought she was a lunatic suggesting I could actually sleep in between all that pain. I sure did it this time around. I'm not sure if I snore when not pregnant but while pregnant, I can definitely make some noise. My moaning was kind of broken so I sounded almost like a bleating sheep. Then the snoring would begin. So it went, "um-mm-mm-mm", sounding like bleating, to snoring, then the bleating would begin and then the snoring again. I wish I had it videotaped.

Some of the contractions found me moaning a bit louder and my mom came over and held my face and spoke to me saying something like, "It's going to be ok". I believe I worried my mom a bit moaning like that because she'd been there for my two previous births and I wasn't as vocal during either of them. Now I knew better. As I moaned my way through each contraction, I imagined myself opening up like a flower blooming, allowing my baby to come forth. At one point I even moaned, "Get oooouuuut" to my baby. Around this time, my midwife asked if she could check me to see how I'd dilated. She asked everyone to guess how far they thought I'd gotten and I wanted to say 8 cm, but I couldn't speak at the time. I heard Orie say "Eight," while others said other numbers. I was 8 cm dilated. It was almost time.

In what seemed like the very next moment, I was feeling the urge to push and was trying to make my way off the couch and to the tub to give birth. My doula, Sabine, stepped right up at this moment. Another word for doula is labor assistant. A doula offers emotional and physical support (and much more) to a laboring woman. No birth should be without one! She held me as I paused for each contraction and rested in between. I held onto her for dear life. One of my favorite pictures from the birth is that of Sabine holding me as I had those last few contractions. She was my rock. After awhile, I started to panic because the contractions were so hard that I had to rest in between them and didn't have much time to take the few steps toward the tub before another one would begin. Plus, the urge to push got stronger. I could feel the baby's head bulging out as I finally got to the rim of the tub. Then I thought, "How on EARTH am I going to lift my leg up to get in?!!?" Then a number of things happened seemingly simultaneously. I remembered my sleeping daughters and asked for them to be brought down for the birth. I remember Sabine being on one side of me supporting me and my husband on the other. My husband started to chuckle and I thought, "What the heck is he laughing about?" then I realized I had a serious death grip on his neck and as soon as I loosened it he laughed and said, "thank you." Poor thing — I was hurting him! Somehow, I got into the tub and squatted just as the girls came downstairs and let out a loud grunt and pushed my big 8-lb 5-oz baby out in 4 minutes! It was a whole lot easier than I thought it would be to push her out.

We thought I was having a boy this time around. You know the whole carrying differently, different kind of pregnancy thing. When the baby came out there was meconium on her genital area. My husband thought maybe it was a boy's scrotum but as it floated away, he winced and then realized that it was another girl!

I was exhausted! I didn't think I'd ever deliver the placenta, I was so tired. After Jasmine came out of there, I wanted my midwife Anne to just yank it out! Thank God I didn't have to get stitches! My husband and Anne helped my second daughter Jenai cut the umbilical cord after it stopped pulsing. Prayerfully, someday, Jasmine will have the opportunity to cut someone else's umbilical cord.

I have never felt more alive than I have while in the process of giving birth. It is truly an awesome experience that I wouldn't want anything — be it another human being, or a synthetic version of what my body naturally produces — to detract from.

Interviews of Birth Attendees

As previously stated, in addition to my husband, I invited my children, mom, and two dear friends, Tori and Orieyama, to attend my homebirth. My mom, husband, cousin, and my oldest attended my birthcenter birth. Of course my mother and husband were present at all three births with my oldest daughter, Jaiela, attended my last two.

Tori has a son, but neither Tori nor Orie had attended a birth so I imagine it was quite an experience for them. I've asked each person to either answer a set of questions or to simply speak about any aspect of the birth they felt inclined to.

My Daughters Jaiela and Jenai

It has occurred to me that my choices in the way I give birth have had profound effects on others, namely my children. At the time of the birth, Jaiela was 9 years old while, Jenai was 3 years old. It came to my attention during a conversation with

Jaiela that she assumed that all children attended the births of their siblings.

If you ask Jaiela, attending her sisters' homebirth was no big deal. She already knew what to expect as she attended her other sisters' birth in 2003. This time, she wanted to catch the baby as she was born but came too late to do so. During prenatal visits, Anne would often joke that Jaiela was going to be a great midwife someday. Jaiela had the ability to feel my belly and be able to tell how the baby was positioned. She was the first person to tell me when she thought the baby moved into a head down position. It turned out she was right because when we went for a prenatal visit, Anne confirmed it. Jaiela could always tell whether the baby jabbed me with a foot, hand or any other body part. It was uncanny how accurate she was at times.

While pregnant with my third, I overheard Jaiela telling someone that she plans to give birth naturally/unmedicated when she is older. Her wish is to either have her first child on a secluded beach or at home. She is happy to have been introduced to birthing this way. Now, when she sees the way the media typically portrays birth, she is able to draw upon her own memory and experiences and knows what birth can be.

Jaiela's only regret was that she didn't come in time to catch the baby. She also wanted to be a part of some of the labor as well, but couldn't stay up. By the time she came, I was in the tub pushing.

Jenai was very happy to be included in the birth. She helped her father cut the baby's umbilical cord. She was very comfortable being a part of it because she'd been thoroughly prepared during prenatal visits. She watched many videos and we read books about preparing for births. Her most memorable moment was when she cut the umbilical cord. She says it made her very happy. Throughout my pregnancy, I referred to the baby as *Jenai's baby* hoping to combat jealousy. I did this with Jaiela when I was pregnant with Jenai. This has worked wonders for us as the girls are very close and care for each other deeply. Jenai is very funny as she attempts mothering a baby that's half her size.

My Mother, Teri

Jaiela was my first grandchild. The labor and delivery of Jaiela were somewhat similar to my experiences in the labor and deliver of her mother, Patrice. I was in labor with Patrice for over 12 hours and had to have a cesarean. Patrice's labor with Jaiela started at 7 a.m., Sunday. Jaiela was born after 2 p.m. on Monday. I stayed with Patrice and Jermaine throughout the labor and subsequent delivery. It was very difficult to watch my daughter having pain that I could do nothing to relieve. After this experience, I was doubtful that my daughter would have another child.

By the time my second grandchild, Jenai, was conceived, Patrice had done her research on alternative birthing methods. She told me she wanted to have the baby at home. I was totally against this for several reasons. First, they were living with me and I didn't want all the blood and mess associated with giving birth in my home. My second concern was if complications developed that required more intensive care. I was also concerned with my daughter being involved in something that I didn't totally understand. There was a lot of tension between us with this pregnancy, and even though I sometimes went with them to the birthing center, I wasn't as involved as I was in the first pregnancy.

On July 3, 2003 my daughter called me at work to advise that her mucous plug had come out and that labor would likely begin soon. While everyone else slept, she and I sat up talking and monitoring her labor pains. This was a very special time for me because the tensions that were present during her pregnancy seemed to evaporate and we were able to rekindle our loving relationship. We were so comfortable that we didn't realize immediately that the pains were coming a little faster and we needed to call the midwife. Thankfully the birthing center was not very far from our home. We arrived at the birthing center at 5 a.m. and our beautiful Jenai was born at 5:18 a.m. Jenai's birth was so very special. I learned more about midwives and experienced the beauty of natural/unmedicated childbirth. It was without the cosmetic approach to this same process that seemed to engulf the hospital birth of my first grandchild, which was also a vaginal but medicated childbirth experience. I was amazed that she got more personal care at the birthing center than with the doctors and nurses at the hospital. The most amazing aspect of Jenai's birth was her resemblance to my deceased father. Over the years she seems to have developed a personality very much like my father's.

On the surface, Jasmine's birth seemed very well planned and structured even though anything could have happened. Patrice had a list of items that she was to collect and had everything readily available on a table near the birthing tub. By now the family had moved into their own home, so Patrice was able to follow her dream of having a homebirth. Since the family was now living out of state, I was not as involved in appointments with the midwife until close to the end of the pregnancy. However, Patrice kept me abreast of everything through phone calls, emails, and pictures. I arrived to help prepare for the birth of Jasmine within days of her proposed delivery date. Jermaine and I pondered over the setup of the birthing tub and worried about possible water leakage from the birthing tub. We also worried that he would be at work and wouldn't get home in time. None of us knew the gender of the baby so this was cause for even more excitement. Finally, labor started! The midwives, Orieyama, and Tori were alerted and seemed to arrive in no time flat. As soon as Patrice was able to make it into the birthing tub, big sisters Jaiela and Jenai were awakened. Jasmine made her grand appearance within minutes to tears and smiles from her grandmother and "aunts" Orie and Tori. The London family was all smiles. Jenai cut the umbilical cord with Dad's assistance for her baby Jasmine. Again, this was learning experience for me. My daughter was able to fulfill her dream of a homebirth with no complications. I was a little unnerved at the beginning of her labor because this baby was a little larger than her previous babies and the midwife had expressed some concern over the size of the baby and a safe delivery. Thankfully our prayers were heard and answered. I have three beautiful granddaughters who are all blessings to our family in their own little special ways. I am extremely grateful for the experience of being present at each of their births.

My Cousin, Tami

I remember the night before Jaiela was born — we were playing Pokeno and keeping track of Trice's contractions. I waited anxiously. We had talked about the possibility of my being in the room; but in the end, I had to stay home. Since I wasn't able to fully experience Jaiela's birth, nothing would keep me from being there for Jenai's.

Jenai's birth was like birth control for me! I swore that if having birth took that much strength, maybe I wasn't the one for it! Jenai's birth was quick. No sooner did they get Trice on the bed, we could see the head. I remember one of the midwives asking me to go get towels. I thought to myself, "I don't know where the towels are, I don't work here!" I looked anyway, and when I got back to the room, I heard this deep groan, like it came from the pit of Trice's belly.

There is a stigma attached to having a baby outside of the four walls of a hospital. Having the option to choose where you want to give birth makes the experience all the more personal and memorable. Some women don't know that they have the choice to choose a method that is still safe and cost effective. I know that if I didn't have pre-existing conditions that made my pregnancies high-risk, I would have opted for a stress-free environment, like a birthing center.

Tori

1. **How did you feel when I invited you to attend my homebirth?**

Wow, I felt honored and excited. I've always wanted to see a live birth. To be able to experience that because of one of my dearest friends made me feel special.

2. **How has the experience changed the way you view birth? How has your view remained the same?**

I view birth very differently now. I think I am too chicken to try and go through a homebirth myself, but I'm hoping to get over that fear by the time I am ready for child number two. However, any woman I see that is pregnant or if conversation comes up about pregnancy, I never hesitate to speak of my experience and ask that they research homebirth and midwifery. My ideas have changed on medicine and how unnecessary many things are that are performed in a hospital during and after childbirth.

3. Were you frightened at any point? Why or why not?

I don't frighten easily, and because I grew up in a family full of nurses, my mind set was to be brave and ready for whatever may happen, good, bad, or scary. During the ride to Patrice's house, I kept thinking "oh my goodness, the time is now," and, once there, waiting for the midwife to get there was the most frightening part. But I tell you, when Patrice's stomach starting to deform and look lopsided, it did make me wonder "What's happening?!!" That was spooky!!!!!!!!!!

4. Are there any particularly memorable moments or feelings you remember from the experience?

Oh man, now I am starting to tear up. To see my friend go through the delivery with absolutely no medication, all I could think about was the type of pain she could be feeling. Outside of her "operatic moaning," I would have thought that she was having no pain at all. Prior to that night, I didn't know too much about homebirth outside of the bits and pieces of information Patrice gave me over the course of her pregnancy. So when I actually saw the aquadoula, which is the birthing tub, I was wondering in what capacity it would be used. But when she climbed in, and Jasmine's head started to come out, I was overwhelmed with watery eyes and feelings of awe and joy. The tears really started flowing when precious Jasmine was fully delivered. Oh man, being that I have gone through childbirth before, I remember how I felt when my son was born, but this feeling was so much greater because it truly looked like a miracle. Especially because I was not the one who did all the work.

The MOST amazing part to me was how alert Jasmine was after being delivered. Her eyes were wide open, she cried just a little, and then was just so peaceful. And she was very alert and awake for some time after. My experience of newborn children is that they are always sleeping, but not Jasmine. It made me wonder are the babies sleeping so much not only because of the stress of being born, but also because of all the medicine that is pumped into the mother's body right before and during delivery.

Then maybe 20 minutes later, after some ohhhhs and ahhhhhhs, the best part I would think for mom, was being in the comfort of her own home. Everyone relocated upstairs to the master bedroom, where mom was nice and comfy in her own home and bed.

I must say, having experienced a homebirth, it definitely has me thinking about having my next child via homebirth. I truly would love to experience it and recommend it to EVERYONE.

Orieyama

I was so excited, first and foremost, because I could be there for Patrice, my best friend and sister. As I drove in the middle of the night worrying and hoping I didn't miss a thing, I thought about how this friendship truly developed full circle and it just wouldn't be right for me not to be there.

I remember the birth of my Jenai and how I received a phone call at 10 a.m. on July 4th. Patrice had been in labor, had gone to the birthing center, and by 5:18 a.m. the baby was born. I just remember her sharing that story with me and feeling so happy for her, but at the same time I felt that I had missed something that I should have been a part of. By the time I saw Jenai and those big eyes with that old soul shining through, I automatically fell in love with her. In fact, she was one of the first babies I had held as a newborn, as I have a great fear of holding new babies. My fear is that I may not know what to do if the baby cries (God forbid!). I know crying is something that babies just do, but I think mothers (which I am not) have some sort of magical powers where as soon as the baby cries they look at their mother and immediately calm down. I did not possess such powers, but with Nai I did. We had an instant bond from the start, which somehow bridged the gap and made me feel that I hadn't missed a thing.

Now was the time for me to conquer my next step in witnessing the beginning of motherhood. That would mean actually being front and center for the birth of the third child, which we just knew would be a boy. I had an even greater fear of participating in such an event. I wasn't sure how much help I would be, how I would behave or if I would be able to withstand watching such an event. I even had visions of passing out from the sight of blood, seeing the head come out, or even witnessing the insurmountable *pain* a mother may endure from a natural birth. I thought it would be devastating. I didn't want to take attention away from my friend having everyone run to my aid when I passed out as she screamed in agony (you can tell I watch a lot of TV, but that was the one and only thing that I had as a reference to childbirth). Whatever the case, I knew that I couldn't miss it and wanted to be there for her in anyway I could.

I realize as I'm writing this that my main fear is *pain*. I fear witnessing pain, feeling pain, and not being able to remedy the problem right away. This was, and still is, where some of my reservations lie in reference to having a child of my own. One would never see me on the side lines holding an anti-children sign, because I do believe that they are the most precious gifts on this earth. I can't think of a better thing to leave behind as your life's legacy than a child. I also know that procreating is what we were made to do and I applaud each and every woman that has experienced it. Understand that, up until now, unlike Patrice I have had terrible cycles filled with pain and discomfort. As of matter of fact, until recent years I would be almost bedridden and just down right sick for no good reason. I always said "If childbirth is any worse than this, you could count me out of those numerous women who make that decision." Ultimately, pain would be the main reason for a childbirth not to occur for me. But I must admit that, after experiencing the birth of Jasmine, it's the end result of holding that child in your arms with "his great looks," and your "girlish grin" that makes you somehow forget about "the horror" and agonizing experience of it all. However, I'm sure that it is all too different when you're the person that has to do those final life altering pushes.

I remember the waiting period and thinking the child was on *his* way for a couple of days. It's funny that, as I look back on this time, she (Jasmine) is as stubborn now as she was a year ago. I guess some traits never leave. We waited for *him* so long that by Friday when I entered the city of Plainfield, walked through the doors, and saw Trice sitting on a gigantic exercise ball, my friend Dana and I were amazed. It was as if nothing changed in the 24 hours that had passed when I last saw her. By then I was even ready for some real action. I guess my fears went out the door. However, I felt like this was the day and I was on Trice's heels even feeling that maybe I should back up a bit. I wasn't quite sure what to do with myself.

When the contractions first began my heart started beating fast. I thought to myself "Breathe deeply." (However, I don't know if that thought was meant for me or Trice, but whatever the case I knew it would help us both.) I didn't think we would ever make it downstairs to the pool. Although I had been educated about the experience, all the knowledge that I possessed went right out the door. I just knew the baby was coming at that moment! I was concerned for my friend as she moaned and vomited, because she is one that would never reveal her day-to-day ailments to anyone. You would not know unless she told you. Admiration comes to mind when I think about how she takes everything in stride.

When we finally got downstairs everyone played musical chairs from the steps to the couch from the couch to the stairs and back and forth to the kitchen. I finally decided to sit on the floor. That's where I felt more grounded. Trice, at the time, seemed to have some major contractions. She would go into some serious moans from deep within, and it would go on for a few minutes and then she'd fall into a deep sleep snoring and everything....like the contractions knocked her out. I chuckled to myself all along, but stayed at the edge of the couch continuing to work on crossword puzzles to bide the time. At one point I remember trying to assist by giving her a cold cloth and I guess it wasn't what she wanted. Next thing I knew, the cloth went flying just missing my head by inches. Normally I would have popped her, but I acquiesced, deciding that she was in enough pain for the moment.

You knew when the contractions were getting closer and more intense. Mama Teresita at one point went into the kitchen and started crying, saying that Trice had never been in this type of pain with the other two children. I consoled her a bit, and said, "Well you know this is the biggest baby she's ever had, too." Not too long after that the moans started turning into outward wailing. Seems like we barely got her from the couch to the pool, but we made it. I ran upstairs and got the children, carried Jenai down the stairs fast, as I knew the moment was near.

All I remember is Trice finally pushing and seeing the crown of the head, the eyes, the whole face, and then I realized that everything was worth the waiting. Tears were rolling down my face as I had never seen such a sight. It reminded me of other times that we are able to take a moment to view God's wonderful works.

Then all of sudden, I hear Nai say, "The baby turned into a girl," as if it happened right before our eyes. I remember having a good laugh.

Everyone went rushing to see the newborn once the cord was cut. I stayed behind knowing that Trice needed more help than the baby. After all, what work was done on Jasmine's part?

This experience showed me that child birthing can be as natural as learning how to walk for the first time. If any type of complication were to have happened, I would not have been able to bear it. I also have to say that if this were Patrice's first child and she decided to have it at home I'm not sure if I would be such a willing participant, but I had much confidence in her beliefs and "tree hugger mentality" as her husband often tells her. She probably would be able to suck me into anything, as she can often persuade the masses. Perhaps I'm not as strong as she and able to tackle such a feat. But when I am blessed with a child, Trice will be the first one there to get me through. I don't know if I will abandon all I've been taught along the way, but, at best, instead of a hospital I'll try a birthing center. Then if there's a second child, we will consider a home birth. You have to crawl before you walk and even Trice had two attempts to get it right on the third time.

My husband Jermaine

I have always been very patient with Patrice and her ideas. If it doesn't sound plain silly (or too drastic) I'm most likely and willing to go along. When Patrice first mentioned homebirth during our second pregnancy, I didn't want to entertain it. It made me feel uneasy. I was definitely one who saw birth as a medical event best left to doctors. The fact that my mother-in-law opposed the idea made me *really* not want to go along. I like to have a back-up plan in place. I wasn't sure there was one for the homebirth until we met with the back-up doctor. That put me at ease.

Another concern with the homebirth was the birthing tub. It is a temperature controlled tub with an aluminum frame and a plastic lining to hold 150 gallons of water. I was afraid that the plastic liner in the tub might somehow rupture and flood our home.

To my surprise the tub was very sturdy and easy to empty after the birth. I was able to use a pump and garden hose to fill and drain it. It was very straightforward and there was no mess made in the process.

The birth center birth with Jenai opened my eyes to what birth could be like outside a hospital and I really enjoyed it. I didn't miss being cramped on a hospital chair or trying to fit into a hospital bed with Patrice as I had endured for 3 days after Jaiela's birth. We were able to go to the birth center, have Jenai, and go home 4 hours later to our own bed. It really makes a huge difference. Even better was the fact that with the homebirth, we never had to leave our home at all.

I could also appreciate being the master of my domain and having everyone else coming in as guests with our homebirth. When something was needed, I was asked about it. In the hospital I felt displaced — as if I weren't needed. Frankly, it all took so long that I ended up sleeping through the majority of the labor. With the homebirth, I was not just a clueless bystander, but very much a part of the entire process. One thing that I (and I suppose any man would have) loved about homebirth is that it is so much cheaper than a hospital birth. Even with it being cheaper, we were blessed even further in that our insurance covered the entire birth in full.

My Final Thoughts

Giving birth at home was absolutely wonderful. It proved to be the perfect alternative to hospital birth. I can't wait to do it again. The experience of giving birth in your own peaceful environment, free of distractions, strangers, machines, and various unnecessary procedures is priceless. I love that Jasmine emerged from the warmth of my womb to the warmth of the aquadoula tub and into my awaiting arms. There were no bright lights, people screaming and scampering about, holding her like a rag doll, pulling here, cutting and wiping there. It was simply peaceful — just as birth should be.

Homebirth Photos

I have included some photos taken by Tori from my home/water birth. My hope is that someone preparing for a birth can share them with their loved ones.

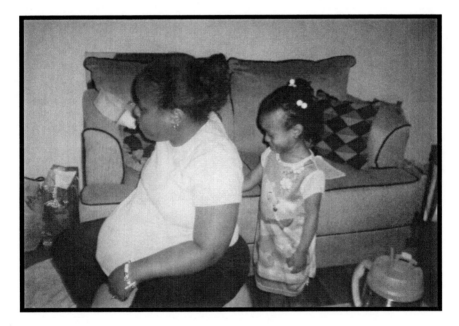

Jenai rubbing my back while I sit on birthing ball

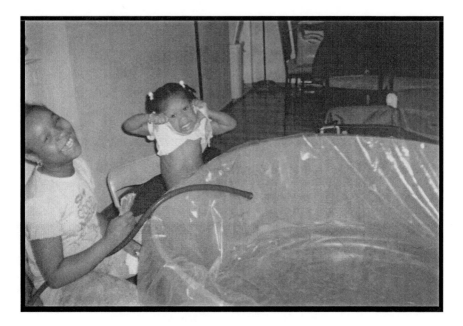

Jaiela and Jenai filling the tub and being silly

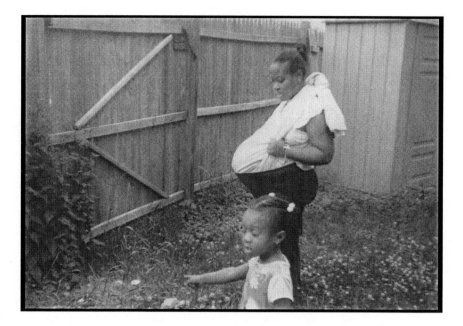

**Using rebozo technique with sheet and looking
at mushrooms in backyard**

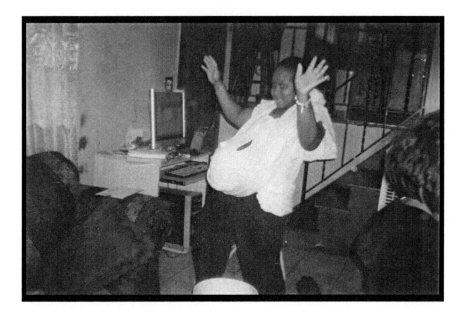

Dancing the baby down while utilizing the rebozo technique

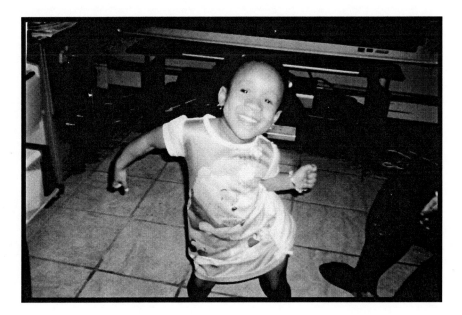

Go Jenai!

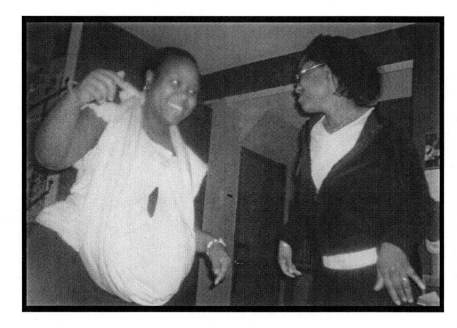

Orie and Patrice dancing

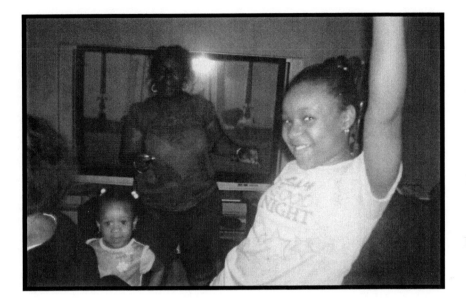

Party over here!

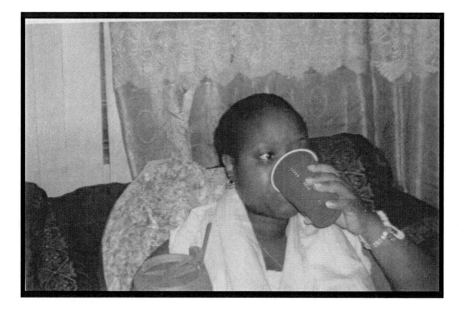

Drinking castor oil

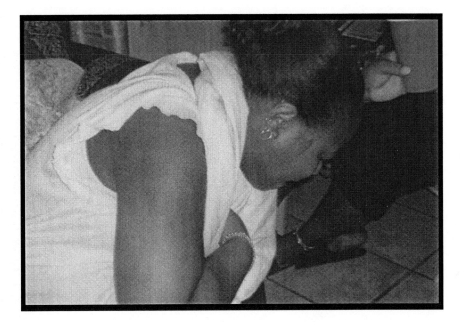

Just after throwing up castor oil

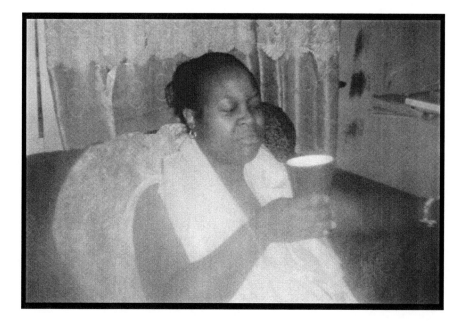

Nasty stuff!

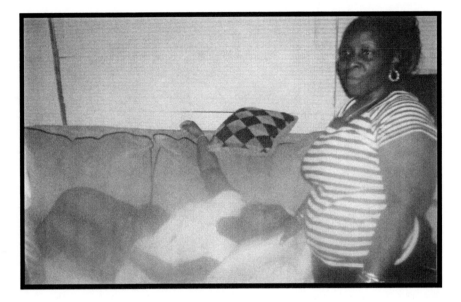

Laboring

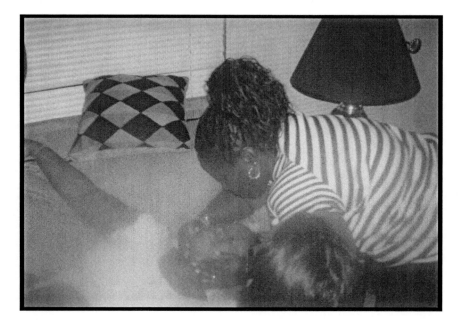

Mom caressing my face

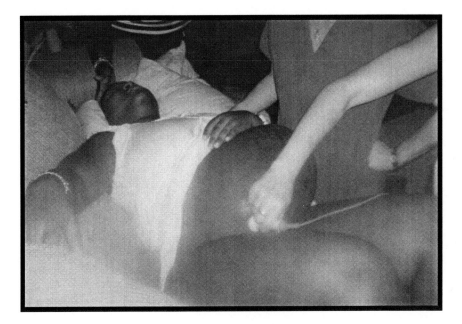

Checking on baby

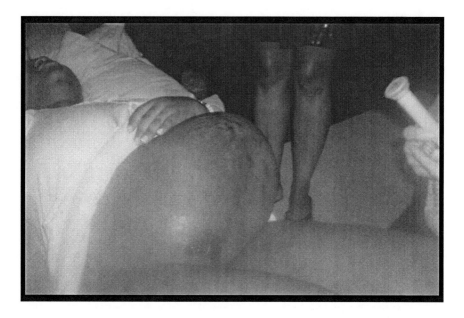

Baby is rotating into the perfect position for birth

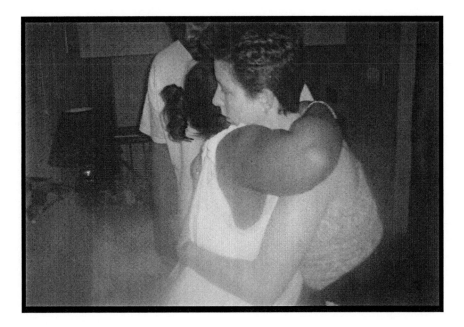

Doula at work

Patrice A. London

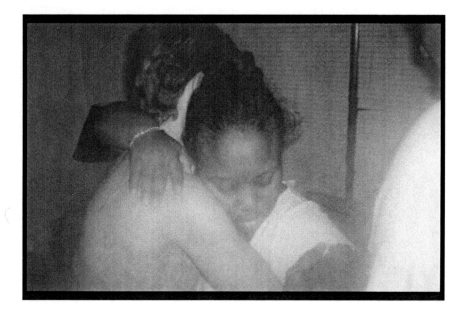

Resting between contractions

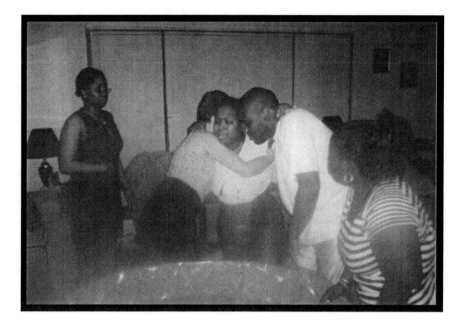

On my way into the tub with Orie and Mom Looking on

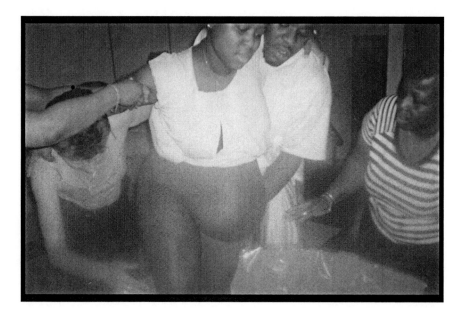

Getting in

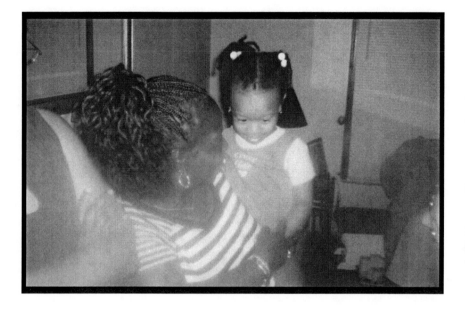

Jenai watching

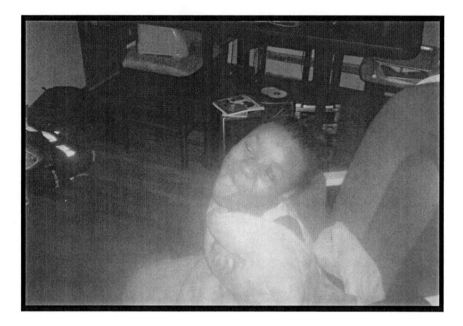

Jaiela being silly

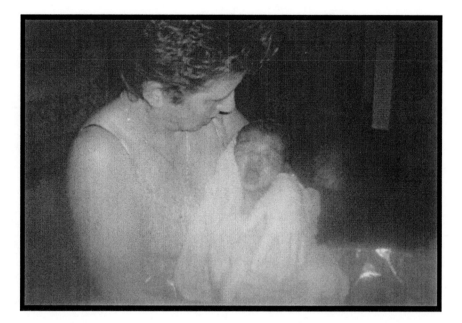

Jasmine is born!

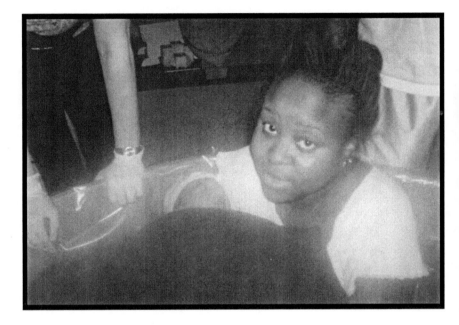

Whew, I did it!

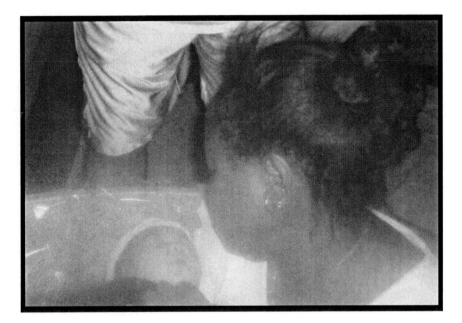

Checking out my new baby

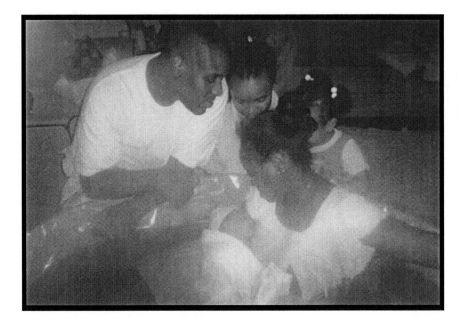

London's huddled around our newbie

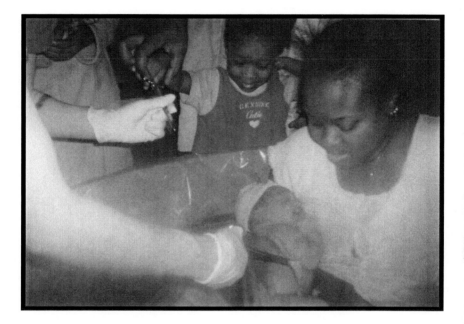

Anne prepares the cord for cutting after it stops pulsing

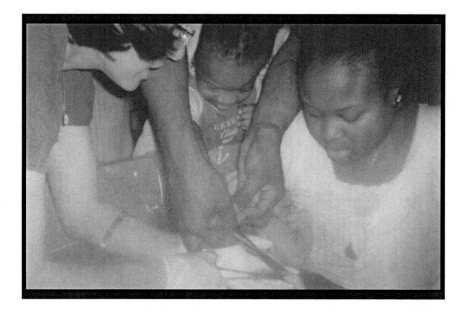

Jenai helps Dad and Anne cut the cord

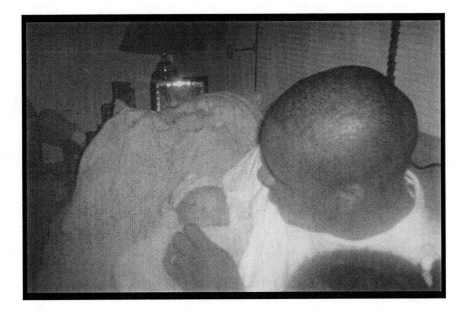

Falling in love with another girl

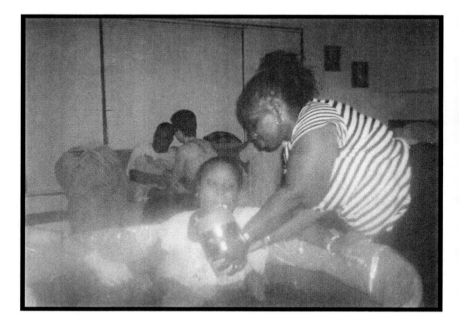

Resting and drinking water

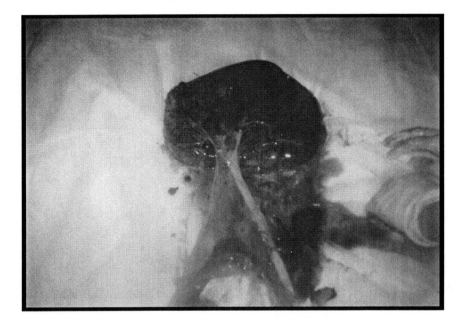

Beautiful placenta that housed Jasmine

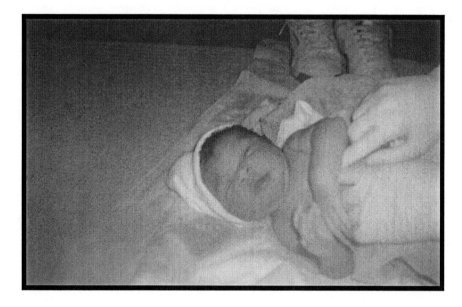

First checkup

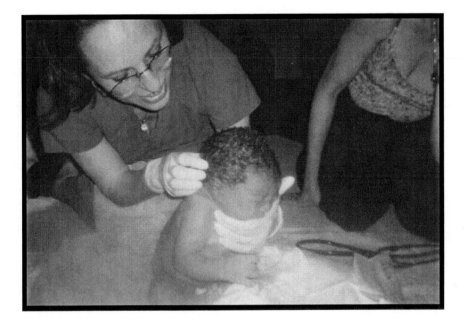

First checkup

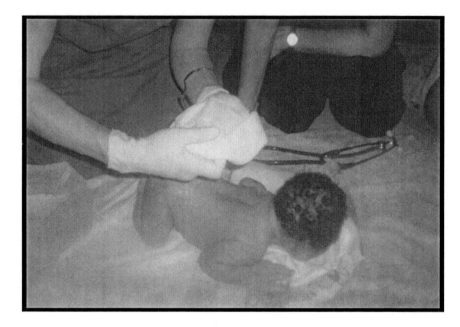

Getting hat

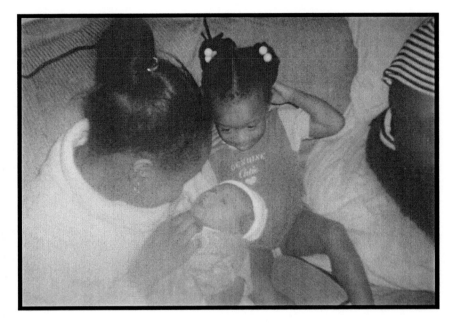

Sisters

Patrice A. London

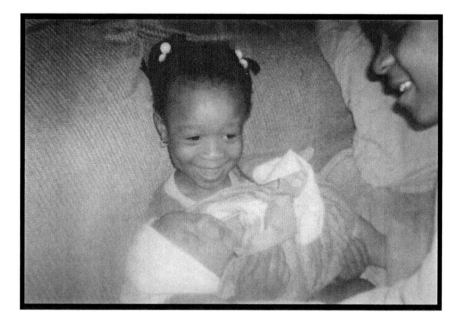

Big sister Jenai

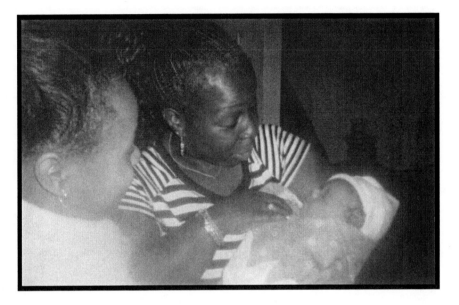

Granny holds Jasmine

Patrice A. London

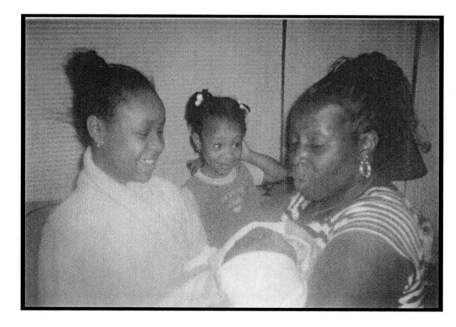

Granny's girls

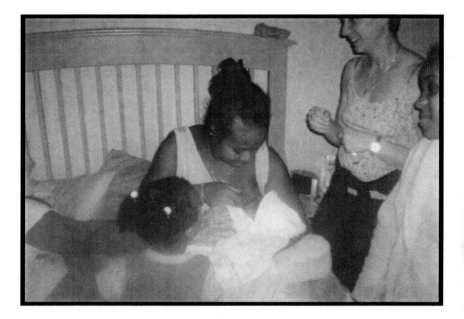

Breastfeeding

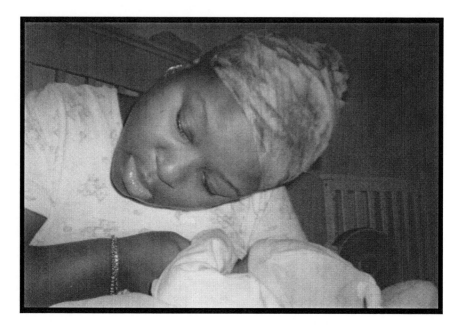

Listening for swallowing

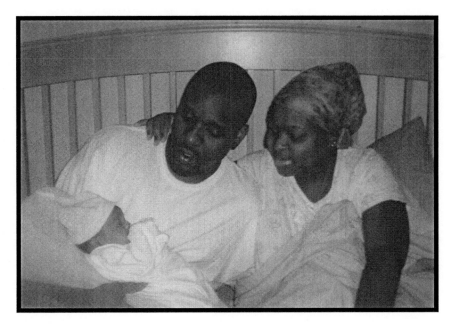

Sleepy but proud parents

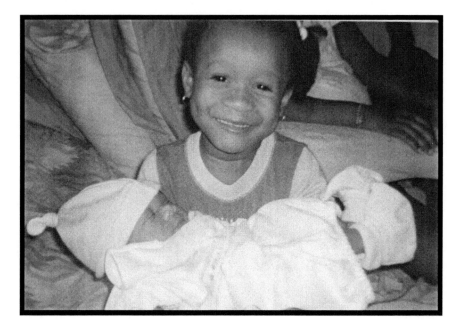

Jenai and Jasmine

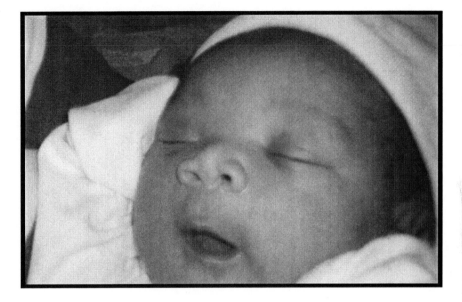

Jasmine Elaine London
June 16, 2007 2:59am

About the Author

Patrice A. London is a native of Washington, DC, and graduate of Duke Ellington School of the Arts (vocal music) and Bethune-Cookman University in Daytona Beach, FL (BA Speech Communication). Patrice currently lives in New Jersey with her husband Jermaine and three daughters, Jaiela, Jenai, and Jasmine. Patrice is a proud Christian Unschooling mother who loves learning alongside her children. Additionally, Patrice is a classically trained coloratura soprano who also loves to sing, act, and write.

Patrice is currently working towards becoming a certified doula, childbirth educator and is excited to be a part of the cast of a play entitled "BIRTH" written by Karen Brody.

LaVergne, TN USA
07 November 2010
203843LV00001B/79/P